UNCOMMON PREGNANCIES

By the Word of God

Dy Wakefield

First Edition, First Printing 2024

Unless otherwise noted, all scripture is from the King James Version of the Bible. [See end of book of Biblical translation]

Limits of Liability and Disclaimer of Warranty
The author and publisher shall not be liable for your misuse of this material. This book is strictly for informational and educational purposes.

Warning – Disclaimer
The purpose of this book is to educate and entertain. The author and/or publisher do not guarantee that anyone following these techniques, suggestions, tips, ideas, or strategies will become successful. The author and/or publisher shall have neither liability nor responsibility to anyone with respect to any loss or damage caused, or alleged to be caused, directly or indirectly by the information contained in this book.

Cover Image: Pixabay

ISBN: 9798335400060

CONTENTS

Prayer

Abba Father, open this reader's eyes, remove the scales so they can see the truth. Open their ears so they can hear the Holy Ghost speak to them in a still small voice. Let the anointing break every yoke, bondage and stronghold. Set them free. Renew their minds. Luke 24:45 states, Then He opened their minds so they could understand the Scriptures. Speak to them in their dreams. Bind confusion. Remove all barriers from them so they can understand. Father, give them wisdom, knowledge and understanding so they can take heed, follow the instructions and do it in Jesus Name.

Reader, allow God to do however he wants to bring manifestation in your life from the subject and content of this book. May this book build your faith so you can act upon it. Hebrews 11:1 AMP states, "Now faith is the assurance (title deed, confirmation) of things hoped for (divinely guaranteed), and the evidence of things not seen [the conviction of their reality—faith comprehends as fact what cannot be experienced by the physical senses]."

Allow God to move on your heart as you read this book. Allow this book to help you, heal you, correct you, mature you, build your faith, get you to your wealthy place and receive what you are believing for.

Please look up the scriptures to get more understanding (Act 17:11).

I want to share the TRUTH that is why this book is heavily worded with the Word of God. Luke 8:12 NIV states, "but the devil comes and takes away the word from their hearts, so that they may not believe and be saved." Satan will try to throw all he can to you to try to stop you from walking in your manifestation. Stand strong and get the word of God in your heart. Make the decision no matter what comes, what circumstance, what situation comes that you will stand on the Word of God until it manifests. Stay in the fight!

Intro

Hello future Mommy,

This book is to be used as a reference of God's word all about conception as you and your spouse are believing for babies. You may have difficulties conceiving (non-infertility issues), infertility or just thinking about conceiving so allow this book to build your faith to conceive.

In your preconception stage you should make a visit with your primary care doctor, OB-GYN, midwife etc. I want to share with you God's perspective according to the Bible with tips in each stage: preconception, pregnancy, birth and lactation. Please meditate on the scriptures listed in the book because it will bring God's comfort and strength to you as well as His wisdom.

God Bless You in your conception in Jesus's Name.

Much Sex, Much More Lovemaking,
Dy

The Promise

Luke 1:13 NIV But the angel said to him: "Do not be afraid, Zechariah; your prayer has been heard. Your wife Elizabeth will bear you a son, and you are to call him John."

Judges 13:3 NIV The angel of the LORD appeared to her and said, "You are barren and childless, but you are going to become pregnant and give birth to a son."

Genesis 18:9-10 ESV 9 They said to him, "Where is Sarah your wife?" And he said, "She is in the tent." 10 The LORD said, "I will surely return to you about this time next year, and Sarah your wife shall have a son." And Sarah was listening at the tent door behind him. 14 Is anything too hard for the LORD? At the appointed time I will return to you, about this time next year, and Sarah shall have a son."

2 Kings 4:16-17 NIV 16 "About this time next year," Elisha said, "you will hold a son in your arms." "No, my lord!" she objected. "Please, man of God, don't mislead your servant!" 17 But the woman became pregnant, and the next year about that same time she gave birth to a son, just as Elisha had told her.

Dy's Vision

December 3, 2022 at 7:25 pm

In a vision I saw an older skinny white female who just died and went to Heaven. As she was standing up there it was revealed to her that she could have had children. This woman wanted children but never had them and as she entered Heaven standing before her she received a message that she could have had them. As I am seeing this the word of the Lord came to me and said "All of the promises of God are Yes and Amen." Sadness came upon me and I wept deeply for her as I prayed in the spirit.

The things which are Impossible with men are POSSIBLE with God. Luke 18:27 KJV

Please, go to my store to purchase a t-shirt, mug, hat, bag and other merchandise with Dy's vision to motivate you to have a baby. https://beautiful-things-by-dy.myspreadshop.com/

The Wife's Vow

1 Samuel 1:11 NIV And she made a vow, saying, "LORD Almighty, if you will only look on your servant's misery and remember me, and not forget your servant but give her a son, then I will give him to the LORD for all the days of his life, and no razor will ever be used on his head."

The Husband's Prayer

Genesis 25:21 NIV Isaac prayed to the LORD on behalf of his wife, because she was childless. The LORD answered his prayer, and his wife Rebekah became pregnant.

Choose the Sex of your Baby

1 Samuel 1:27 NLT I asked the Lord to give me this boy, and he has granted my request.

1 Samuel 1:20 NLT and in due time she gave birth to a son. She named him Samuel, for she said, "I asked the Lord for him."

John 16:24 NIV Until now you have not asked for anything in my name. Ask and you will receive, and your joy will be complete.

Psalm 37:4 NIV Delight yourself in the LORD and he will give you the desires of your heart.

Preconception

Judges 13:3-5 KJV 3 And the angel of the Lord appeared unto the woman, and said unto her, Behold now, thou art barren, and bearest not: but thou shalt conceive, and bear a son. 4 Now therefore beware, I pray thee, and drink not wine nor strong drink, and eat not any unclean thing: 5 For, lo, thou shalt conceive, and bear a son; and no razor shall come on his head: for the child shall be a Nazarite unto God from the womb: and he shall begin to deliver Israel out of the hand of the Philistines.

This is the stage where you began preparing for your pregnancy. You would consider your health situation such as your weight, your eating conditions, then how to prepare your body to conceive and carry your baby or babies full term.

In the above scripture the Angel was preparing this woman with a mandate for pregnancy not to drink alcohol and abstain from certain food.

Future mom in the Preconception stage it's all about getting your body healthy and ready to conceive and birth a healthy baby. There are two elements in this, You and Your baby.

Here are five (5) items to consider just so your personal research. These are only suggestions so pray about it.
   1. **Exercise**
        o   Consider aerobic exercises.
        o   Consider lifting weights.

2. Eating
- ○ Consider the Weston A Price eating plan for Preconception, Pregnancy and Lactation.

3. Supplements
There are many supplements out there that are beneficials to preconception, pregnancy, after birth and lactation. Here is a list to consider in your personal research.
- ○ Consider your Microbiome so probiotics and prebiotics are important
- ○ Consider Beef Liver pills as a new prenatal choice
- ○ Consider Higher quality prenatal multivitamin with Folate instead of Folic Acid
- ○ Consider Methylfolate
- ○ Consider Inositol
- ○ Consider Omega-3s with DHA
- ○ Consider Cod Liver Oil
- ○ Consider Vitamin D with vitamin K2

4. Beauty
- ○ Consider your beauty products (skincare, makeup, hygiene products and fragrance) be mindful of the chemicals in them such as Endocrine Disruptors.

5. Environmental
- ○ Consider EMF (Electric and Magnetic Fields) and get protected.

These five (5) items are just for you to consider so your own personal research. These are only suggestions so pray about it.

Pregnancy

Ruth 4:13 NIV So Boaz took Ruth and she became his wife. When he made love to her, the Lord enabled her to conceive, and she gave birth to a son.

Genesis 21:1-2 TLB Then God did as he had promised, and Sarah became pregnant.

Genesis 30:22 NIV Then God remembered Rachel; he listened to her and enabled her to conceive.

Exodus 2:1–2 NIV 1 Now a man of the tribe of Levi married a Levite woman, 2 and she became pregnant and gave birth to a son.

2 Kings 4:17 But the woman became pregnant, and the next year about that same time she gave birth to a son, just as Elisha had told her.

This is the fun stage of sex, sex, sex, enjoying lovemaking, your husband's body and your body embracing the creation of your baby or babies.

Ooo La La!!!

Praise God for His Promise

Luke 1:49 KJV For he that is mighty hath done to me great things; and holy is his name.

1 Samuel 1:26-28 KJV 26 And she said, Oh my lord, as thy soul liveth, my lord, I am the woman that stood by thee here, praying unto the Lord. 27 For this child I prayed; and the Lord hath given me my petition which I asked of him: 28 Therefore also I have lent him to the Lord; as long as he liveth he shall be lent to the Lord. And he worshipped the Lord there.

Stress Free Pregnancy

Proverbs 14:30 AMP A calm and peaceful and tranquil heart is life and health to the body.

1 Peter 5:7-8 KJV 7 Casting all your care upon him; for he careth for you. 8 Be sober, be vigilant; because your adversary the devil, as a roaring lion, walketh about, seeking whom he may devour.

Colossians 3:13 MSG Quick to forgive an offense. Forgive as quickly and completely as the Master forgave you.

John 14:27 KJV Peace I leave with you, my peace I give unto you: not as the world giveth, give I unto you. Let not your heart be troubled, neither let it be afraid.

2 Timothy 1:7 KJV For God hath not given us the spirit of fear; but of power, and of love, and of a sound mind.

1 John 4:18 KJV There is no fear in love; but perfect love casteth out fear: because fear hath torment. He that feareth is not made perfect in love.

Hebrews 4:9-11 NIV 9 There remains, then, a Sabbath-rest for the people of God; 10 for anyone who enters God's rest also rests from their works, just as God did from his. 11 Let us, therefore, make every effort to enter that rest, so that no one will perish by following their example of disobedience.

To have a stress free pregnancy you must position yourself to live a life of stress free. You may no longer answer calls from those complaining family and friends. You may no longer have to answer the door as well to keep them out. You have your space and you need that space to be stress free. You focus on what you can control.

Steps toward a stress free life:
- Sex with your spouse
- Sleep
- Pray
- Laugh. Proverbs 17:22 KJV A merry heart does good, like medicine.
- Forgive
- Repent
- Support Group i.e. Spouse, friends
- Bible Reading
- Praise God
- Focus
- Think of things lovely and pure. Philippians 4:8

Midwife

Exodus 1:17,19-21 NIV 17 The midwives, however, feared God and did not do what the king of Egypt had told them to do; they let the boys live. 19 The midwives answered Pharaoh, "Hebrew women are not like Egyptian women; they are vigorous and give birth before the midwives arrive." 20 So God was kind to the midwives and the people increased and became even more numerous. 21 And because the midwives feared God, he gave them families of their own.

Choosing a Baby Name

27

Luke 1:13 NIV But the angel said to him: "Do not be afraid, Zechariah; your prayer has been heard. Your wife Elizabeth will bear you a son, and you are to call him John.

Luke 1:31 NIV You will conceive and give birth to a son, and you are to call him Jesus.

Judges 13:24 NIV The woman gave birth to a boy and named him Samson. He grew and the LORD blessed him.

Genesis 21:3 KJV And Abraham called the name of his son that was born unto him, whom Sarah bare to him, Isaac.

Choosing a name is very important because of the meaning. In the Bible a man named Jabez was a victim of being named wrongly because it affected his life negatively. Jabez is living in a curse because of his name.

Jabez's name means sorrow, pain and painful delivery.

Think about that as you read
- 1 Chronicles 4:9 KJV And Jabez was more honourable than his brethren: and his mother called his name Jabez, saying, Because I bare him with sorrow.
- 1 Chronicles 4:9 NIV Jabez was more honorable than his brothers. His mother had named him Jabez, saying, "I gave birth to him in pain."

To break the curse Jabez sought the Lord: 1 Chronicle 4:10 KJV And Jabez called on the God of Israel, saying, Oh that thou wouldest bless me indeed, and enlarge my coast, and that thine hand might be with me, and that thou wouldest keep me from evil, that it may not grieve me! And God granted him that which he requested.

Here are some names in the Bible with great meaning: Genesis 17:5 NIV No longer will you be called Abram; your name will be Abraham, for I have made you a father of many nations.

Abraham's name means "Father or many nations."

Genesis 17:15-16 NIV 15 God also said to Abraham, "As for Sarai your wife, you are no longer to call her Sarai; her name will be Sarah. 16 I will bless her and will surely give you a son by her. I will bless her so that she will be the mother of nations; kings of peoples will come from her.

Sarah's name means "Mother of many nations."

Choosing a baby name is important. You could bring a blessing or curse on your baby by the name you give.

When to Announce Pregnancy

Hebrews 11:23 NLT It was by faith that Moses' parents hid him for three months when he was born. They saw that God had given them an unusual child, and they were not afraid to disobey the king's command.

Luke 1:24 NASB Now after these days his wife Elizabeth became pregnant, and she kept herself in seclusion for five months.

Luke 1:36 NIV Even Elizabeth your relative is going to have a child in her old age, and she who was said to be unable to conceive is in her sixth month.

Luke 1:56 NIV Mary stayed with Elizabeth for about three months and then returned home.

This is your special moment and as you read in the above scripture some of those women waited three months, five months, six months. This is your time, don't be pressured by family members or friends.

Nurture your Baby Soul in while in the Womb

How to properly nurture your baby's soul in the womb? is by being mindful of your words and actions. Especially how you and your spouse communicate. Because baby's pick up emotions of their parents that can either cause or prevent baby soul wounds.

Psalm 147:3 NIV He heals the brokenhearted and binds up their wounds.

According to John Loren Sanford, "We have a mind in our spirit before we have a brain. And that in the mind of our personal spirit we can experience, react rightly and wrongly to what we perceive as happening around us, happening in the womb, happening in our parents, happening in our family, happening in the world so that we can come out of the womb already wounded. Already disposed in certain directions which may be wrong for us." (Core)

He continues to say, "If a father and the mother have a good life together, good prayer life, good understanding, they're united and they're love play is holy and clean and good. That brings no harmful effects to children in the womb. We found that people who have been raised by parents who have it together. They don't have valence and hurts and wounding, prenatally from what their parents did in making love to each other while they were in the womb. But if the parents are, don't have it together, are fighting or committing lust with one another you know that you can commit lust with your own spouse. if you use the other person for your gratification without respect to cherish the other for the others sake you're committing lust with your own spouse. And when that has happened that can wound a child in the womb." (Core).

Talk to your baby in the Womb

"Around 18 weeks of pregnancy, your little one hears their very first sounds. By 24 weeks, those little ears are rapidly developing. Your baby's sensitivity to sound will improve even more as the weeks pass. The limited sounds your baby hears around this point in your pregnancy are noises you may not even notice. They are the sounds of your body. These include your beating heart, air moving in and out of your lungs, your growling stomach, and even the sound of blood moving through the umbilical cord." (Timmons).

Jeremiah 1:5 NIV Before I formed you in the womb I knew you, before you were born I set you apart; I appointed you as a prophet to the nations.

Psalm 139:13 TLB You made all the delicate, inner parts of my body and knit them together in my mother's womb.

Psalm 139:14 KJV I will praise thee; for I am fearfully and wonderfully made: marvellous are thy works; and that my soul knoweth right well.

Psalm 139:15-16 ERV 15 You could see my bones grow as my body took shape, hidden in my mother's womb. 16 You could see my body grow each passing day. You listed all my parts, and not one of them was missing.

Psalm 119:73 NIV Your hands made me and formed me.

Full term Pregnancy

Luke 1:57 KJV Now Elisabeth's full time came that she should be delivered; and she brought forth a son.

Genesis 25:24 KJV And when her days to be delivered were fulfilled, behold, there were twins in her womb.

Easy Labor and Delivery

Isaiah 66:7 NIV Before she goes into labor, she gives birth; before the pains come upon her, she delivers a son.

Luke 2:7 ESV And she gave birth to her firstborn son and wrapped him in swaddling cloths and laid him in a manger, because there was no place for them in the inn.

Ruth 4:13 NIV and she gave birth to a son.

1 Samuel 1:20 NLT and in due time she gave birth to a son.

Genesis 38:27 NKJV Now it came to pass, at the time for giving birth, that behold, twins were in her womb.

Circumcision

Luke 2:21 NIV On the eighth day, when it was time to circumcise the child, he was named Jesus, the name the angel had given him before he was conceived.

Genesis 21:4 NIV When his son Isaac was eight days old, Abraham circumcised him, as God commanded him.

Breastfeeding

Isaiah 66:11 NIV For you will nurse and be satisfied at her comforting breasts; you will drink deeply and delight in her overflowing abundance.

Genesis 21:7 NIV And she added, "Who would have said to Abraham that Sarah would nurse children?"

Luke 11:27 NIV As Jesus was saying these things, a woman in the crowd called out, "Blessed is the mother who gave you birth and nursed you."

Milestones

Isaiah 65:20 ERV In that city there will never be a baby who lives only a few days.

Luke 2:40 NLT There the child grew up healthy and strong. He was filled with wisdom, and God's favor was on him.

Judges 13:24 NIV The woman gave birth to a boy and named him Samson. He grew and the LORD blessed him.

Well Baby Check

Psalm 139:16 ERV You could see my body grow each passing day. You listed all my parts, and not one of them was missing.

Weaning

Genesis 21:8 KJV And the child grew, and was weaned: and Abraham made a great feast the same day that Isaac was weaned.

1 Samuel 1:22 NIV Hannah did not go. She said to her husband, "After the boy is weaned, I will take him and present him before the LORD, and he will live there always.

SHAMELESS PAST

Abortion

You had an abortion and maybe more than one. You feel shame. You think God is punishing you. You think you will never have a child because you had an abortion. You may say, "I killed a child, why would God bless me with another one."

You have been condemned by religious people about the sin of having an abortion they gave you scriptures such as:
- Proverbs 6:17 KJV A proud look, a lying tongue, and hands that shed innocent blood.
- Proverbs 1:16 KJV For their feet run to evil, and make haste to shed blood.
- Exodus 20:13 KJV Thou shalt not kill.

<u>BUT</u>

Galatians 3:13 NKJV Christ has redeemed us from the curse of the law, having become a curse for us (for it is written, "Cursed is everyone who hangs on a tree").

You can be free be healed and made whole and begin a new life in Christ and God can and will bless your womb.

You feel unworthy! Jesus died on the cross for that shame and gave you worth.

Go to the **Prayer for FREEDOM of Shame** to become free, healed and whole. THEN allow God to use your womb to bring in His heritage.

Psalm 127:3 KJV Lo, children are an heritage of the LORD: and the fruit of the womb is his reward.

Drugs

53

You were a drug user. You feel shame. You think God is punishing you for your past and He would not trust you with having a baby even though you are drug free.

You have been condemned by religious people about the sin of having an abortion they gave you scriptures such as:

- Titus 2:12 KJV teaching us that, denying ungodliness and worldly lusts, we should live soberly, righteously, and godly, in this present world.
- Galatians 5:20-21 GWT 20 idolatry, drug use, hatred, rivalry, jealousy, angry outbursts, selfish ambition, conflict, factions. 21 envy, drunkenness, wild partying, and similar things. I've told you in the past and I'm telling you again that people who do these kinds of things will not inherit the kingdom of God.

<u>BUT</u>

Galatians 3:13 NKJV Christ has redeemed us from the curse of the law, having become a curse for us (for it is written, "Cursed is everyone who hangs on a tree").

You can be free be healed and made whole and begin a new life in Christ and God can and will bless your womb.

Go to the **Prayer for FREEDOM of Shame** to become free, healed and whole. THEN allow God to use your womb to bring in His heritage.

Psalm 127:3 KJV Lo, children are an heritage of the LORD: and the fruit of the womb is his reward.

Prostitution

You used to prostitute in your past. You have got out of that life. But you feel shame. You think God is punishing you for your past..

You have been condemned by religious people about the sin of having an abortion they gave you scriptures such as:
- 1 Corinthians 6:16 NIV Do you not know that he who unites himself with a prostitute is one with her in body? For it is said, "The two will become one flesh.
- Leviticus 19:29 NIV Do not degrade your daughter by making her a prostitute, or the land will turn to prostitution and be filled with wickedness.
- Deuteronomy 23:17-18 NIV 17 No Israelite man or woman is to become a shrine prostitute. 18 You must not bring the earnings of a female prostitute or of a male prostitute into the house of the Lord your God to pay any vow, because the Lord your God detests them both.
- Ezekiel 16:33-NIV All prostitutes receive gifts, but you give gifts to all your lovers, bribing them to come to you from everywhere for your illicit favors.

<u>BUT</u>

Galatians 3:13 NKJV Christ has redeemed us from the curse of the law, having become a curse for us (for it is written, "Cursed is everyone who hangs on a tree").

1 Corinthians 6:17 NIV But whoever is united with the Lord is one with him in spirit.

Go to the **Prayer for FREEDOM of Shame** to become free, healed and whole. THEN allow God to use your womb to bring in His heritage.

Psalm 127:3 KJV Lo, children are an heritage of the LORD: and the fruit of the womb is his reward.

Parents Guilt

Parents, Single Moms, Single Dads, Older parents you are holding guilt and shame in your life because you didn't have good prenatal care. Maybe you didn't know you were pregnant and missed out on getting the nutrients. Your baby now has a defect. Your baby lacks in an area because of that. Yes, that includes the father who didn't follow prenatal care. You didn't know the importance on your side. You may have thought it was all on the mother.

Now mother and daddy you feel guilt, shame because your baby, your child or even your adult child is suffering from that conception.

Today the guilt and shame STOPS in Jesus's Name. Your baby, child or adult child doesn't have to suffer anymore because of Jesus.

I don't care if you are 80 years old and have a 60 year old child and because of the lack of knowledge of nutrients they are still suffering from the lack of knowledge of prenatal care.

Mom, dad maybe you missed it on the first baby and got the nutrition knowledge on the next babies and they are in perfect health. So you feel guilty about your first born and even your child holds hate towards you.

BUT FREEDOM, HEALING & WHOLENESS HAS COME TO YOU ALL TODAY.

Psalm 139:13-16 MSG Oh yes, you shaped me first inside, then out; you formed me in my mother's womb. I thank you, High God—you're breathtaking! Body and soul, I am marvelously made! I worship in adoration—what a creation! You know me inside and out, you know every bone in my body; You know exactly how I was made, bit by bit, how I was sculpted from nothing into something. Like an open book, you watched me grow from conception to birth; all the stages of my life were spread out before you, The days of my life all prepared before I'd even lived one day.

I bind lies from your mind for thinking God created your child to be like that. The devil is a liar.

Go to the **Prayer for FREEDOM of Shame** to become free, healed and whole. THEN allow God to use your womb to bring in His heritage.

Psalm 127:3 KJV Lo, children are an heritage of the LORD: and the fruit of the womb is his reward.

Prayer for **FREEDOM** of Shame

I will be addressing eight scenarios to pray for you mommy, daddy and your baby, or now he or she is a child or now an adult child. If you all could read this together it would be great. But if not you can stand in for the rest of the family. If you are standing for your family just call out their names now.

Scenario one, due to having an abortion.

1 John 1:9 If we confess our sins, he is faithful and just to forgive us of our sins and cleanse us from all unrighteousness

You must confess your sins to God tell Him say, "Abba Father I confess I aborted a baby (babies) and I repent of that lifestyle. I receive my forgiveness and cleansings.

Scenario two, due to having an abortion as a Christian.

Maybe you are a Believer or Christian and you got an abortion as a Christian and you are feeling double guilt, shame and condemnation. God is love and Jesus died for your sins to cleanse you of it. He took your sins on His body on that cross.

You must confess your sins to God tell Him say, "Abba Father I confess I aborted a baby (babies) and I repent of that lifestyle. I receive my forgiveness and cleansings.

Scenario three, due to drug use.

Matthew 6:13 KJV And lead us not into temptation, but deliver us from the evil one

You must confess your sins to God tell Him say, "Abba Father I confess I used drugs and I have no desire for it. I repent of that lifestyle. I receive my forgiveness and cleansings. If there is any dormant desire, demons in my soul hidden for the desire for drugs I am asking you to wash me clean so it will never come up. I know through tragedy like Covid the fear and stress people went back to drugs. I despise drugs and I renounce it to be completely whole in Jesus Name."

Scenario four, due to prostitution.

Hebrews 11:31 NIV By faith the prostitute Rahab, because she welcomed the spies, was not killed with those who were disobedient.

You must confess your sins to God tell Him say, "Abba Father I confess of being a prostitute, call girl, sex worker, or escort. I despise it. I have no desire for it. I repent of that lifestyle. I receive my forgiveness and cleansings. I ask to be free and whole to bring in a generation free from this curse. I receive my forgiveness and cleansing in Jesus Name."

Scenario five, due to nutrient negligence the baby has a birth defect.

John 9:2-3 His disciples asked him, "Rabbi, who sinned, this man or his parents, that he was born blind?" Neither this man nor his parents sinned," said Jesus, "but this happened so that the works of God might be displayed in him."

Abba Father in Jesus Name I command Your hand on the mama, the daddy, the baby, or if he or she is a child or an adult now to break the curse off them. Forgive the parents of ignorance in regards to the lack of prenatal care. Heal them so they can forgive themselves. Jesus, remove the guilt and shame.

Abba Father now I command your hand upon the baby, or if he or she or they are a child now or even an adult child heal them their soul and body and make them whole. According to Matthew 15:30 And great multitudes came unto Jesus, having with them those that were lame, blind, dumb, maimed, and many others, and cast them down at Jesus' feet and He healed them.

Scenario six, the mama and daddy you may have been born without prenatal nutrients so it's time for you to be healed as well. This would almost be like a generational curse that will continue through the generational line unless stopped.

Say this mama, daddy, child or adult child, "I receive the healing power of Jesus I receive my body heal and whole. I forgive myself. I forgive my parents for their ignorance in lack of prenatal care. Jesus, blood removes the shame and guilt and I receive His healing power."

Reader, I reverse the curse off you and soak your soul with the Power of the Cross and Resurrection, the Blood of Jesus, Dunamis Power, Glory Light of Jesus and Holy Ghost Fire. Producing Excellent of Soul.

Scenario seven, due to sin it's the cause of birth defects, psychological and learning disabilities as well as baby soul wounds.

Acts 3:2 And a certain man lame from his mother's womb was carried, whom they laid daily at the gate of the temple which is called Beautiful, to ask alms

To the mama and daddy Jesus died on the cross for everyone's sins and for you to be healed and made whole. To get to that place of freedom you will need to repent so if any of the following situations are yours then I need you to repent to remove the shame. I will be listing four areas of different sins to repent for but if you do not see it listed but you have a conviction in your heart from the Holy Ghost exposing what you should repent for then repent of it now.

One, if the mama aborted the baby but the baby lived in the womb. Two, if the daddy was doing drugs, adultery, porn, a prostitute, a one night stand, he raped her and she became pregnant. Three, if the mama was doing drugs, adultery, porn, a prostitute, a one night stand when you got pregnant. These will cause physical, emotional and spiritual ramification on your child. You may have gotten saved since then but there is guilt. I want to add number four, this other area even though it is not a sin on the mother's part because she was raped the man who raped her can cause these ramification on the baby also the trauma from the mother who was raped. All these cause rejection in the baby during conception. They feel rejected in the womb and once born and even grow up as a child to an adult their life is moved by that rejection. And you may now think you have a troubled child but its soul wounds from birth. Rejection makes them feel not wanted, they may get into drugs, have an affair, confused about their sexuality, learning problems and so much more.

Say this, "Father, I repent of all my sins, omission and commission. I receive my forgiveness and cleansing. I also repent for the sins that caused others not to be able to fulfill their purpose, calling, assignments, and destiny in Jesus Name."

Say this, "Father, I renounce all acts of the flesh."

The Holy Ghost will reveal anything else you need to repent of, who else you need to forgive and what else you need to renounce as you grow in God.

Scenario eight, to the mama and daddy maybe you were born by those situations so it's time for you to be healed as well.

Say this, "Father, I forgive all those who have sinned against me including my parents for their sins against me and after forgiving them I bless them and release them to you. I forgive myself. Jesus, blood removed the shame and guilt and I receive His healing power."

Reader, I reverse the curse off you and soak your soul with the Power of the Cross and Resurrection, the Blood of Jesus, Dunamis Power, Glory Light of Jesus and Holy Ghost Fire. Producing Excellent of Soul.

I know you may be emotional, you could be crying, it's the anointing breaking bondage off you. Lord show this listener Your glory. You are being healed and delivered supernaturally. Your body is being healed. I want you to do the impossible move that body part that you were having issues with. If you have a limp walk, if you have pain check it, if you have a growth or rash check it. If you can't jump, jump. Do what you couldn't do before. If you have an addiction, notice that desire is gone. Notice the shame gone. Take an Act of Faith by walking, moving, checking to see.

You will notice demons leaving your body, you are being set free, you are being healed, the shame and guilt is leaving. You will experience vomiting, you may burp, cough, yawn, you may have to pee a lot, you will feel weights coming off your shoulders, necks, head. You may feel like your spirit is leaving your body but it's not your spirit it's demons. You may feel like you have a head cold, sinus or eye pressures, and feel dizzy. I bind you demons from trying to cut them as you exit. Come Out Now no dramatic show. I cast you to the lake of fire in Jesus Name. Enter no more in this listener or their family in Jesus Name.

If you like to be a part of the Family of God all you have to do is say "Jesus, I want you to be my Lord and Savior. I believe God raised you from the dead. I renounce satan and all his devices."

If you like to be baptized in the Holy Spirit to speak in tongues just say, "Holy Ghost I desire that gift and I receive it thank you." The Holy Ghost will guide you in this beautiful language that will bring you intimately to God. Holy Ghost loose this listener's tongue.

Games

All games are created by Dy Wakefield

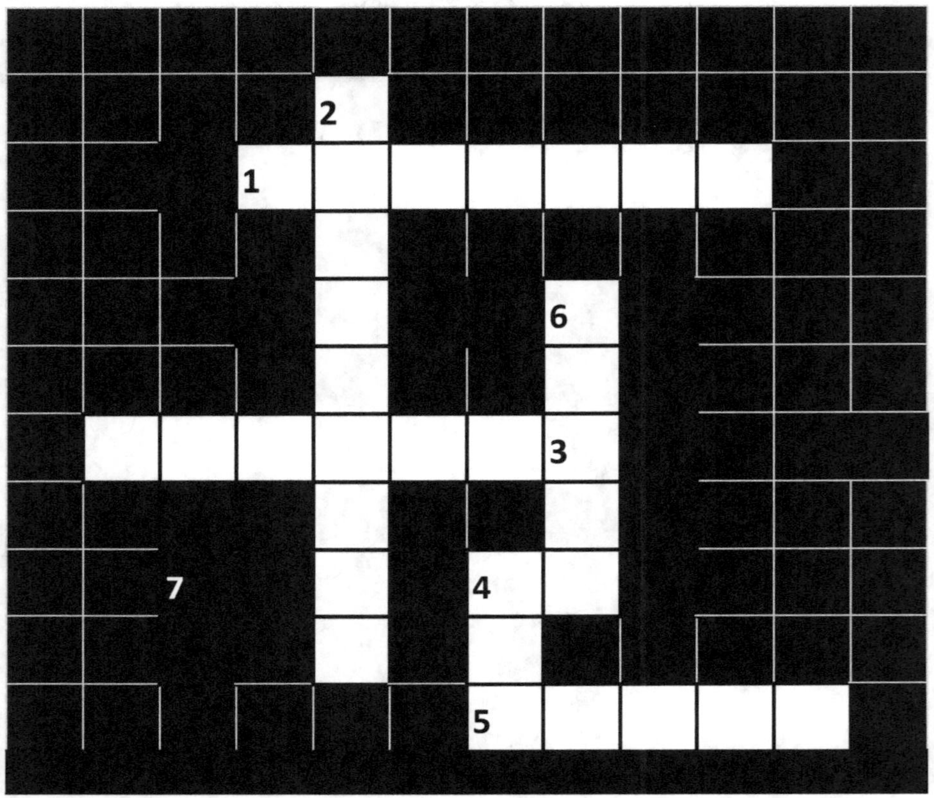

Across

1   God's guarantee
3   God's Supernatural manifestation
5   Male parent

Down

2   Another name for Gestation
4   Another name for Abba Father
6   Female parent

A	B	C	D	E	F	G	H	I
6	2	21	17	20	11	16	19	23

J	K	L	M	N	O	P	Q	R
8	10	14	26	9	25	15	12	22

S	T	U	V	W	X	Y	Z
18	1	7	4	13	3	24	5

7	9	21	25	26	26	25	9

15	22	20	16	9	6	9	21	24

2	24		16	25	17	18

13	25	22	17

Answers

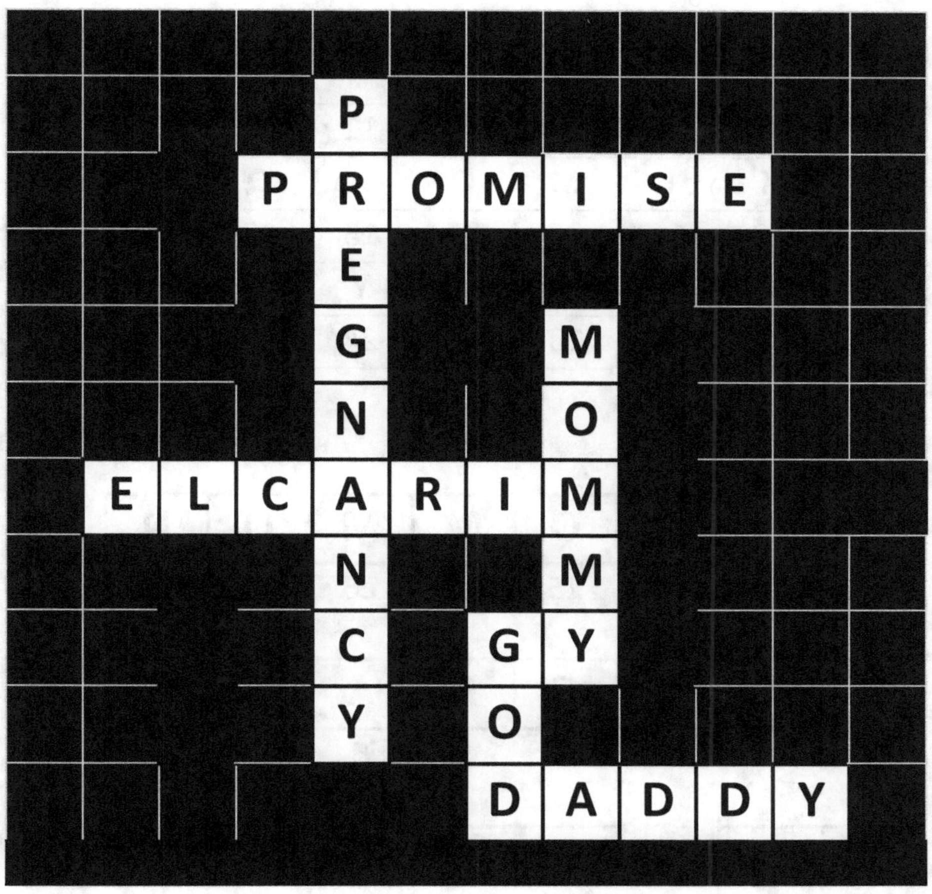

P
PROMISE
PREGNANCY
MOMMY
ELCARIM
GY
GOD
DADDY

A	B	C	D	E	F	G	H	I
6	18	21	17	20	11	16	19	23

J	K	L	M	O	P	Q	R	S
8	10	14	26	25	15	12	22	2

T	U	V	W	X	Y	Z
1	7	4	13	3	24	5

U	N	C	O	M	M	O	N
7	9	21	25	26	26	25	9

P	R	E	G	N	A	N	C	Y
15	22	20	16	9	6	9	21	24

B	Y
2	24

G	O	D	S
16	25	17	18

W	O	R	D
13	25	22	17

Free Materials

~ENGLISH~

Be Fruitful and Multiply
https://bit.ly/3zLy5hW

I AM a Mother
https://bit.ly/3zKIx9r

~ESPAÑOL~

Sean Fructíferos y Multiplíquense
https://bit.ly/3S8M1bW

Soy Madre
https://bit.ly/3Wsh2JB

~AMAZON purchases~

Supernatural Miracle Pregnancy: Covenant Promises of God
https://a.co/d/exoSh1M

Embarazo Milagroso Sobrenatural: Pacto Promesas de Dios
(Spanish Edition)
https://a.co/d/awqAKwt

References

Core Bible Study. (2015, March 14). *Ministering to Prenatal Wounds* [Video file]. YouTube.
https://youtu.be/qyaZlSsamnk?feature=shared

Timmons, J. (2018, January, 5). *When can a fetus hear?* Healthline.com
https://www.healthline.com/health/pregnancy/when-can-a-fetus-hear#1. Accessed August 7, 2024.

In Closing...

Immerse yourself in the scriptures in this book. Receive healing, wholeness, freedom and an Open Womb to bring forth God's heritage.

Psalm 127:3 KJV Lo, children are an heritage of the LORD: and the fruit of the womb is his reward.

Be Blessed!!

About the Author Dy

Dy Wakefield, The Queen of Wealth Advice™ is an Advisor, Multi-Genre Author, Multi-Social Entrepreneur, Speaker, and Aviation Enthusiast.

<u>BUSINESS CREDENTIALS</u>
In 2020 God inspired Dy to transition to Advisor so she took her seat on her Royal Throne.

She was the founder of the now defunct companies Wealthy Woman Dy Investments, Inc., Dy Wakefield International, LLC., Empowering You Events, LLC. Two Biblically Sexually Explicit companies Pleasure Your Husband and Pleasure Your Wife. She was also 51% share partner in Oglesby Concrete Specialists, LLC.

She has written over 100 books and you can check out her Amazon Author Page where she was blessed to use Amazon publishing as a tool to help her become an author and be creative experimenting in many different genres.

Dy also had four radio shows: The Wealthy Woman Dy Morning Show, Pleasure Your Husband Radio, Pleasure Your Wife Radio and Comfort & Hope in the Midst Radio.

Dy has over 20 years in Accounting, Bookkeeping, Tax Preparations, Business Start-Up and Notary Services. Dy received her BS in Accounting from Clemson University and a Master in Finance specializing in Financial Planning from Kaplan University now Purdue University Global.

Queen Dy's passion for helping women stemmed from personal experience of being underpaid and underappreciated in Corporate America. She wants to break the cycle by helping birth out leaders. 'Dy' is the acronym for "delivery" and she calls herself the midwife for business women. Being a double minority Black and Woman, Dy at times felt like she was at the bottom of the totem pole but she knows that it is God's grace and faith that elevate you not what society has limited you. None of the Higher Education she received compares to the WISDOM she receives from GOD it surpasses all.

Dy's foundation is God because through her many failures. God allowed a "Whale" in her life, this is in reference to Jonah and the Whale, which was used to stop her from continuing on the wrong path and pivoting her to the Way of Success. This led her to forever depend on God and be obedient to whatever He asks her to do, say and go. Basically God allowed LIFE to kick her #@!? She is now able to instill WISDOM of success upon you.

DY'S VISION

To Teach, Empower, Train and Create over a Million Wealthy Business Queens to be financially independent and to use their businesses to Impact Communities Globally and Fund the GOSPEL.

PURPOSE/MISSION

Dy has dedicated her life to Empower Women by **Awakening the Queen inside** to be Leaders to own businesses and to be world changers. To help them achieve their destiny through a balanced life and excellence.

Dy has dedicated her life to Empower Wives by **Awakening the Sexual Prowess inside** for their husbands, 1 Corinthians 7:3 NLT version states the husband should Fulfill his Wife's Sexual Needs. God has given Wives' Sexual Needs. There is an inner Sex Vixen that you haven't tapped into. It's your feminine nature to be turned on. Sex & Sex Drive is a Gift from God so "Sex is not dirty it's Pleasurable." Sex is to be enjoyed by both satisfying each other's needs. Ooo La La! You came into a covenant with God and your husband so it's not an emotional thing but a mutual agreement to shake them sheets on a continual basis.

This is a sisterhood to **TEACH. EMPOWER. TRAIN. CREATE** to be Wealthy and Healthy. A focus on the importance of balance in **FAITH, FAMILY, FITNESS, FINANCE and FUN** as women embrace the role of Queen ruling and reigning in their business Queendom.

Acknowledgments

To God Be the Glory (God, Jesus & the Holy Ghost)

BIBLE ORDER:

<u>Get Your House in Order</u>

Spouse 1st, children 2nd, The Rest & Me time 3rd, The Purpose, Assignment & Destiny 4th as God is the Center of your life.

Give

The one who is taught the word [of God] is to share all good things with his teacher [contributing to his spiritual and material support]. Galatians 6:6 AMP

If you were blessed by the teaching in this book Galatians 6:6 states that you can give to the teacher.

Please pray to God if He would like for you to give and if He says yes then ask Him how much you should give.

If you are giving, please wrap your faith with your giving. Your faith is what you have been meditating on, scriptures, from this book. **As you give, say "I receive."** Make notation of your giving.

I speak over your giving. "May God bless you with a hundredfold in Jesus Name." I thank you for the gift, I receive it and God Bless You.

Ways to Give:

https://transformativebeautybydy.weebly.com/give.html

https://www.paypal.com/donate/?hosted_button_id=2QSP84WT9K3GW

<u>Other Ways to Give:</u>

Paypal
email: BeautybyDy@yahoo.com
Cash App $BeautybyDy8
Money Gram   Beauty by Dy
Western Union   Beauty by Dy

<u>Personal Gifts to Dy</u>
(i.e. birthday, honor, etc.)

Paypal   paypal.me/QueenDyWakefield
Cash App $DyWakefield
Venmo   @DyWakefield
Zelle   prosperdy@yahoo.com
Google Pay   Dy Wakefield

CRYPTOCURRENCY:
Bitcoin   @DyWakefield
Ethereum   @DyWakefield
USD Coin   @DyWakefield

Contact

Website: https://transformativebeautybydy.weebly.com/

Social Media
Facebook: www.facebook.com/DyWakefield
X: https://x.com/DyWakefield
Instagram: www.instagram.com/DyWakefield
YouTube: www.youtube.com/@dywakefield
YouTube: www.youtube.com/@dythequeen

Send Testimonies to email:
whereveryousetfoot@yahoo.com

Miracle Healing and Deliverance Prayer

Abba Father in Jesus Name I call you as Jehovah Rapha the God who heals and as Jehovah Mephalti the God who delivers. I command your hand to stretch forth upon this reader. Father, release your healing, miracles, signs, wonders, and deliverance angels. Holy Spirit, fall right now wherever the reader is and heal and cure them.

Reader, the anointing of God will come upon your head to your feet and saturate your body, heal you and minister to you. The anointing will go in your body and destroy the yoke of bondage making the infirmities, sicknesses, diseases, pain, addictions leave. Lay hand on that part of the body and call out the issue its name because it has to bow in Jesus Name.

I demand every cell, bones, organs and tissues in your body to line up with the Word of God. I bind every demon and cast them out to the lake of fire. Some will leave because of the anointing but the others won't because you are giving them permission to stay.

Reader, you need to renounce those demons inside of you to be set free, don't keep some and get rid of the rest. Totally surrender to the anointing and let them all go by saying, "I renounce all demons and blood covenants. I sever ties from them and the people I am wrongly involved with." .

I bind the spirits of Jannes and Jambres. I bind messengers of satan, seducing spirits, doctrines of devils and infirmity spirits. I bind all and any forms of witchcraft, clairvoyance, and astral projecting that was done to you. I bind all and any forms of witchcraft off this reader and their family.

Reader, right now call out a family member, loved one, spouse, child, friend etc.

Abba Father release your vengeance and return every curse sent upon the reader back to sender 100-fold. I call fire from Heaven upon satanic altars with the reader's pictures, names, addresses, DNA samples, clothing, effigies, voodoo dolls of their image. Let the blood of Jesus nullify that. I bind and break curses sent with words "over my dead body" and return it back to the sender. I bind and cancel all demonic dreams such as recruiting, monitoring, mind controlling, mind reading, evil eye, entering in demonic partnerships, contracts, marriages, blood covenant, creating demonic spiritual babies and children with demons, sexual activity, perverse activities, paralysis. I bind and cancel demonically infiltrating music, miscarriages, sterileness, birth defects, premature deaths, fears, sicknesses and diseases through dreams. I bind demonically administering drinks, food, foreign substances, drugs, etc. in dreams.

Jesus, transcend back to the reader as a baby in the womb and heal the soul wounds.

I bind all demons and I loose them back to the sender bringing great fear, great dread, great tremble and great torment upon the sender and then I cast the demons to the lake of fire. I decree the wealth of the wicked "the sender" will come to the reader in Jesus Name.

Be healed, be made whole, **RESTORE** in Jesus Name. New body parts come! Creative Miracles come!

****

To those who are missing body parts due to birth, surgery, mutilation, injury etc).
Body Parts Restore!!!!

Matthew 15:30-31 KJV [30]And great multitudes came unto him, having with them those that were lame, blind , dumb, **maimed {missing body parts}**, and many others, and cast them down at Jesus' feet; and he healed them: [31]Insomuch that the multitude wondered, when they saw the dumb to speak, **the maimed to be whole {restored body part}**, the lame to walk, and the blind to see: and they glorified the God of Israel.

****

Reader, now I want you to do the impossible, move that body part that you were having issues with. If you have a limp walk, if you have pain check it, if you have a growth or rash check it. If you couldn't jump, jump. Do what you couldn't do. If you have an addiction, notice that desire is gone. Take an Act of Faith by walking, moving, and checking to see.

Deliverance:

There's another step to deliverance and it's about you repenting of your sins and forgiving those who hurt you. Holy Spirit, reveal the sins they need to confess so they can be cleansed of it.

Holy Ghost, reveal to them those they need to forgive. Reader, it may be hard to forgive so you have to ask Jesus to give you that spirit to forgive. You are <u>only</u> forgiving those people through confession to God, you are not going to them and saying I forgive you, you heathen. Your forgiveness is a release from that hurt, a form of bondage holding you trapped in your life. Receive the Times of Refreshing from the Lord Acts:3:20.

Start here in your confessions:
- Abba Father, I repent of (state the sins) I receive my forgiveness and cleansing in Jesus Name.
- Abba Father, I forgive (state their names). I bless them and I release them to you in Jesus Name.

Abba Father I soak this reader's soul with the Power of the Cross, the Power of the Resurrection, the Blood of Jesus, the Dunamis Power, the Glory Light of Jesus, the Holy Ghost Fire, the Fire of God and Thundering of God in their soul producing Excellence of Soul. Whom the Son makes free is free indeed John 8:36. God cut them free from the cord of wickedness Psalm 129:4.

PLEASE NOTE: Healing can come instantly or gradually. Your part is to thank God for your healing.

WARNING:
Don't stop your medicines until you get checked by your doctor to get the documented proof.

Covid Prayer

{*Put your hand on your heart*}. Father right now the name of Jesus I curse any and all forms of Trauma in their lives in Jesus Name, any and all forms of Stress and the effect of stress on their life I command every bit of it to go in Jesus Name. Father right now in the name of Jesus I command the Immune System to be healed, whole and strong in Jesus Name. I speak Endorphins into their body to kill off any form of stress hormones in Jesus Name. I curse any Prions in their body in Jesus Name. I command the PH Balance to be restored to normal in Jesus Name. In Jesus Name no sickness, disease or virus can come into your body. {Put your hands a little lower} in Jesus Name I command all Hormones to go into perfect harmony and balance in Jesus Name. Hallelujah! Hallelujah.

If you've had either Covid or the Vaccination because both have poison in them. So Father right now in the Name of Jesus I send the word of healing to each person that fits in either one of those categories right now in the name of Jesus. I curse any Prions that have been injected into your body whether through the virus or other means. I curse all of that in the name of Jesus. Any side effect of either one of those I command it to be gone in Jesus Name. I speak new lungs in Jesus Name. New Immune System in Jesus Name. No inclination for Blood Clots. And any form of Chronic Fatigue Syndrome I command all of that to go and the Brain Fog that comes with it, comes with both of them. So the brain fog I command all of that to go in Jesus Name. Centered, the mind restored in Jesus Name. Thank you Jesus. Amen.

Reference: 12/27/2021 "Festival of Miracles 2021" at David Herzog Ministries's Apostolic Center in Chandler Arizona. Joan Hunter prayed the above prayer and commissioned everyone to go and pray this prayer for people.

Salvation

If you're tired of trying to do things your way in life, how about giving Jesus a try? Ask Jesus to be the Lord and Savior over your life surrendering all to Him. Allow Him to come into your heart. Be sincere. Be fed up with how your life is going now and tell Jesus you are ready to receive Him, His love, protection, help, deliverance and healing. All I ask is for you to just try Him, your life will never be the same.

Say this, "Jesus, come into my heart, I am tired of living the life I am living now. I confess that you died on the cross for my sins and rose again by the Holy Spirit. I renounce satan and all his devices. Jesus, I choose you to be the Lord and Savior over my life."

To the Believer who finds yourself far from the truth I bind deception and I loose clarity. Don't feel condemned, Jesus still loves you. He died for you. Come back into the Father's loving arms. Please repent so your sins will be blotted out so that the "Times of Refreshing" will come.

I just want to acknowledge that God sent Jesus the Messiah the Chosen One for you. When you confess your sins to God, your sins are washed away by the blood of Jesus. He is no longer angry with you if you accept this Gospel message.

Please as a Help and Warning: Do not step your foot into any church until you hear from God. He may have you attend a church online. Do not be led by friends or family, be led by the Holy Ghost and join the church to get your spiritual food to grow.

Salvation for Priests called as Kings (Queens)

To Pastors, Priests, Ministers, Apostles, Prophets, Teachers and Evangelists who are **not saved** who never accepted Jesus as your Lord and Savior. Do So Now! This is no longer a career profession for you. This is no longer a financial venture for you. This is no longer controlling the strings "the minds of people." **Repent God says Repent.** God is cleaning up His church and the leadership positions. Confess to God! Repent and turn from your wicked ways. He has a leadership position for you in BUSINESS!

If you will indeed judge yourself, you shall not be judged. As you seek My face and desire to be cleansed by Me in all truth and sincerity of heart, I will judge you in the secret place, and the things that are in the secret place of your heart shall not be made manifest to others. I will do it in the secret place, and no man will know it. The shame that will be seen on many faces shall not be seen on your face. Therefore in mercy and love, I am instructing you in order that you may partake of My glory. As you are willing to walk with Me and rejoice in your sufferings, you shall in turn partake of My glory. Look unto Me, for you have need of power to overcome the wicked one and the bondage in other's lives. ~Prophet Stanley Frodsham

2 Peter 3:9 NLT The Lord isn't really being slow about his promise, as some people think. No, he is being patient for your sake. He does not want anyone to be destroyed, but wants everyone to REPENT.

God says "Come out from that position you are in and Come into the Marketplace where I called you for business."

God says, "Come out from among them and get in your rightful position as King / Queen."

Repent and turn to God and allow the Holy Ghost lead you into the Destiny God has for you where He can bless you physically, spiritually and financially.

Accept God's will and forsake yours because if you keep fronting standing in a leader position that God didn't call you to He will close that door on you to your **SHAME.**

Say this, "Jesus, come into my heart, I am tired of living the life I am living now. I confess that you died on the cross for my sins and rose again by the Holy Spirit. I renounce satan and all his devices. Jesus, I choose you to be the Lord and Savior over my life."

1 Samuel 3:12-14 NLT [12]I am going to carry out all my threats against Eli and his family, from beginning to end. [13]I have warned him that judgment is coming upon his family forever, because his sons are blaspheming God and he hasn't disciplined them. [14]So I have vowed that the sins of Eli and his sons will never be forgiven by sacrifices or offerings.

Preach the Gospel in your Business that God called you to.

Baptized in the Holy Spirit

PLEASE NOTE: You must be saved or in other words you must have accepted Jesus Christ as your Lord and Savior by confessing that with your mouth before you can be baptized in the Holy Spirit.

ACTION STEP

If you like to be Baptized in the Holy Spirit with the ability of speaking in tongues Say this: "Holy Ghost I desire that gift of Speaking in Tongues and I receive it thank you."

The Holy Ghost will guide you in this beautiful language that will bring you intimately to God.

Holy Ghost loose this reader's tongue.

God as Your Business Partner

Your business is not where you want it to be, how about giving Jesus a try? Do you know there are many business people in the Bible? In the Old Testament there is Abraham, Issaac, Jacob, Job, Boaz all had business in agriculture plus many others including women. In the New Testament the disciples Peter, James, John and Andrews were all fishermen, Matthew a tax collector, Apostle Paul a tentmaker plus many others including women.

Make a decision today to allow God to take over and help you increase abundantly so you can enjoy the fruits of it with your family. Allow Him to lead you to prosper (teach you to profit Isaiah 48:17).

Say this: "Jesus, I choose you to be the Lord over my businesses so God I am asking that You, Jesus and the Holy Ghost be my Business Partners."

As a Business Partner God can direct you in the right products and services, right pricing levels for your products and services, who to hire and who not to hire, who to fire, who to have as clients or who not to deal with. God can reveal things to you that you cannot discern with your eyes. Let God lead you and watch Him accelerate your business.

Repent for Wrong Business Practices

NOW Queen if you have been doing wrong business practices in your businesses it's time to get right. Get right with God. Abba Father, remove the scales from this Queen's eyes so she can see and know truth.

Queen, pray this prayer:

"Father, I repent for doing and allowing wrong business practices in my businesses I stop today. I take full responsibility for my actions and my employees. I receive my forgiveness and cleansing. Father, you are all knowing and omniscient so I ask you to be my business partner. I will be led by your spirit, the Holy Spirit as You download ideas, concepts, solutions, and witty inventions through Him to me. I will give you glory in all I do in Jesus Name. I forgive myself and I receive your love. I will be led by the Holy Ghost to remove the dishonest practices from my businesses in Jesus Name."

Queen don't trip, we all make mistakes we all have lived for that DOLLAR you are on the right track now. You no longer have to work hard for that DOLLAR watch God show you how to multiply to create millions with ease and have balance in your life.

Say this decree daily:
I know who I serve! Abba Father in Heaven! Hallowed be thy Name!™

A prophetic decree from Dy's dream on July 25, 2024 at 10:33 am
Read my book: "God or Mammon:Where is your Allegiance?

Show Your Commitment

Think about committing to giving financially to God trusting Him with your Business by honoring Him back because what you commit to God He will bless.

As believers you accepted Jesus as your Lord and Savior so that means you are Abraham's seed according to Galatians 3:29. Abraham gave tithes to Melchizedek see Genesis 14:18-20. Abraham gave tithes before the law. We are not about the law but of Grace which is Jesus our High Priest. Just make slight changes switching from Malachi 3 tithe to Hebrews 4 & 7 tithing to the High Priest Jesus Christ. Action Steps: 1. Prepare your tithes at home 2. Lift it up towards Jesus 3. Say, "Lord Jesus, I present my tithes to you as my High Priest." (If you are married, do this together). 4. Then give your tithes in your church collection plate.

Your money is important so you need to know if it is going into **GOOD GROUND**. If you are thinking of your church to give to you better make sure the ground is good. You may have to ask your Pastor if he or she is saved, is Jesus your Lord and Savior? You may have to ask the Pastor if he or she gives in the collection plate? You may have to ask your Pastor if he or she has a side chick or side dick? Seek the Holy Ghost and He will lead you into all truth. Because God's house should be Holy and it starts with leadership. If you find yourself doing those wrong things, check the leadership of your church.

One thing to remember, do not forget that God is the one that gave you this wisdom and enablement (Deuteronomy 8:18). Praise God in all you do. Always share your testimony to others of the Goodness of God in your life.

Spend time with God

1. Designate 30 Minutes Daily
2. Preferably first thing in the morning (wake up earlier if you have to)
3. Avoid your cell phone, internet, etc. (unless it is needed)
4. Take 5 minutes and enter the presence of God with Singing, Thanksgiving and Praise (Psalm 100)
5. Take 5 minutes and just sit and listen for God (be quiet and listen)
6. Take 5 minutes journal what you are hearing and seeing
7. Take 10 minutes read a chapter a day start with Proverbs the wisdom book
8. Ask God what does that chapter pertain to you
9. Take 5 minutes to pray
10. You are honoring God and He will accept this so yes set a timer you will not offend Him.
11. Take Communion.

Global Business Queens Support

https://www.globalbusinessqueens.com/support.html

I am asking for **supporters** on a continuous basis to support my **Global Vision** to Empower Women in Business. There will be projects, events, traveling and so much more in the making. Be inspired by the free teaching materials on the website and the social medias that it may bring success in your life.

Dy's vision:
To Empower, Train and Create over a Million Wealthy Business Queens to be financially independent and to use their businesses to Impact Communities Globally and Fund the GOSPEL.

Each month I will email you a Business & Empowerment MP3 and monthly letter to empower you in your business or start-up and for personal encouragement. Also, via email I will let you know what projects, events and traveling I am doing and its updates. **You will be informed of what we've done, what we are doing and what we're going to do.** You will always be in my DAILY prayers. **Thank you, you're beautiful!** I will not take this investment lightly because you work hard for it.

Thank you again for supporting "The Cause" your giving will (1) support ministries that train and educate others to be Business Owners. Empowering and Training (2) women prisoners and former inmates to become Business Owners and (3) Global Reach.

Awake O Queen, from slumbering! Arise, and sit on your throne to decree.™

~ Dy Wakefield

Queen Dy is a Charitable Queen

Eight (8) Philanthropic areas of Empowering Women and Girls (born as a female and has a womb) Genesis 1:27, Genesis 5:2

Our Global Division
Women's Economic - support entrepreneurship, community impact and funding the Gospel. *(Revelation 5:10, Luke 10:33-34, 1 Timothy 6:18)*

Our United States Division
Women's Health – eradicating infertility and obesity, supporting healthy living naturally through mindset change, nutrition, nutrients and exercise. *(Isaiah 54:1, Psalm 128:3, Exodus 23:26, Deuteronomy 28:4, Exodus 1:19, Isaiah 66:11, Proverbs 23:2, Romans 12:2, Genesis 1:29-30, Genesis 9:3, 1 Corinthians 6:19, 1 Corinthians 9:27)*
Women's Education - support accredited, post-secondary institutions in South Carolina Clemson University and Southern Wesleyan University *(Luke 6:40, John 8:31, Matthew 28:19, Daniel 1:4)*
Women in the Arts - support fashion, etiquette, literature, performing arts, media arts, and visual arts *(Genesis 1:27, Exodus 36:1, Exodus 35:31-33, Exodus 31:3, 1 Thessalonians 4:11, Deuteronomy 28:12, Psalm 68:11)*
Women's Protection - support eradicating modern slavery, women prisoners transition and domestic violence shelters *(Isaiah 61:1, John 8:36, Isaiah 42:7, Psalm 91)*
Women with Guns - support and honor women in the military, women working in the field of homeland security, women forest rangers, police women and women first responders *(Romans 13:3-4, 1 Peter 2:13-14)*
Women who Fly - supporting organizations that encourage Women in Aviation *(Isaiah 60:8, Proverbs 3:23 MSG, Isaiah 58:14)*
Women in Sports - supporting Women in Sports *(1 Corinthians 9:27, Philippians 3:14, 1 Corinthians 9:24, Isaiah 40:3)*

Faith • Family • Fitness • Finance • Fun

Decree of "Now"

If you laid down your dream, you know, that business, that ministry, those dance shoes, that baby, that ball, that tool, pick it up.

Pick it up I say, Pick it up!

You are in the Spirit of Now.

Now I can have that Business.
Now I can have that Missions Ministry.
Now I can Dance.
Now I can have that Baby.
Now I can play Pro Basketball
Now I can be a Mechanic
Now! Now!

Say Now and Pick it Up!

Decree over your life! Decree that whatever dream you let die or put aside that you pick it up Now. Decree you will get goals for it. Decree you will find a mentor to help you. Decree over your life!

- Dy Wakefield

What We Believe

Don't get it Twisted our Loyalty is to God, Jesus and the Holy Ghost

James 1:8 NLT Their loyalty is divided between God and the world, and they are unstable in everything they do.

1. The Father, The Son & The Holy Ghost
2. God The Creator
3. We Are The Image Of God
4. God Created Male And Female
    a. Genesis 1:27 NLT So God created Human Beings in his own image. In the image of God he created them; male and female he created them.
5. God Created Marriage
6. Covenant Between God And Man
7. Babies Are A Gift From God
8. Jesus's Death And Resurrection
9. Jesus As Our Living Epistle
10. The Holy Ghost Our Helper
11. Jesus's Death And Resurrection
12. Jesus As Our Living Epistle
13. The Holy Ghost Our Helper
14. The Bible: [Our Foundation]
15. The Gospel: [How We Share]
16. Faith
17. Discipleship
18. Long Life
19. Wealth And Health
20. Capitalism:
    a. Deuteronomy 8:18 NIV But remember the Lord your God, for it is he who gives you the ability to produce wealth, and so confirms his covenant, which he swore to your ancestors, as it is today.
21. Support Israel
22. Impact Communities & Fund The Gospel

CHOOSE LIFE

Deuteronomy 30:19

When you make a decision to 'Choose Life' you are deciding to Live and Be Blessed. If you decide to choose the other way you are deciding to Die and Be Cursed. To make it easy for you. God is saying 'CHOOSE LIFE'.

Choose Life to live and fulfill your destiny on earth! Don't give up on life by choosing the other alternative. There is a vision inside of you that must be fulfilled. Choose to follow your purpose!

Other Biblical translations

New International Version (NIV) Holy Bible, New International Version®, NIV® Copyright ©1973, 1978, 1984, 2011 by Biblica, Inc.® Used by permission. All rights reserved worldwide.

Living Bible (TLB) The Living Bible copyright © 1971 by Tyndale House Foundation. Used by permission of Tyndale House Publishers Inc., Carol Stream, Illinois 60188. All rights reserved.

New Living Translation (NLT) Holy Bible, New Living Translation, copyright © 1996, 2004, 2015 by Tyndale House Foundation. Used by permission of Tyndale House Publishers, Inc., Carol Stream, Illinois 60188. All rights reserved.

New American Standard Bible®, Copyright © 1960, 1971, 1977, 1995, 2020 by The Lockman Foundation. All rights reserved.

Easy-to-Read Version (ERV) Copyright © 2006 by Bible League International

The Message (MSG) Copyright © 1993, 2002, 2018 by Eugene H. Peterson

New King James Version (NKJV) Scripture taken from the New King James Version®. Copyright © 1982 by Thomas Nelson. Used by permission. All rights reserved.